Desk Pilates
Living Pilates Every Day

Angela Kneale, OTR
Occupational Therapist
Certified Pilates Instructor

Desk Pilates
Living Pilates Every Day

Copyright 2008 by Angela Kneale, OTR

Published by:

OPTP
Tools for fitness, Knowledge for health
3800 Annapolis Lane, Suite 165
Minneapolis, Minnesota 55447
800.367.7393
www.optp.com

Printed in the United States of America

Cover and Interior Design: Steve Bubb
Photography: Dewey Koshenina
Photography Producer: Dani Hartmann
Pilates Models: Kara Petta, Carlton Morris, Christy Lyons
Editors: Susanne Schaars, MSPT, Dip.MDT, Patricia Rouner Morris

ISBN 0-9799880-3-9

Every effort has been made to ensure that the information contained in this publication is accurate and current at the time of printing. The ideas, exercises, and suggestions are not intended as a substitute for consulting with your health care provider. All matters regarding your health require medical supervision. Neither the author nor the publisher shall be liable or responsible for any loss, injury, or damage allegedly arising from any information or suggestion in this publication.

Consult your physician or health care provider before starting any type of physical exercise.

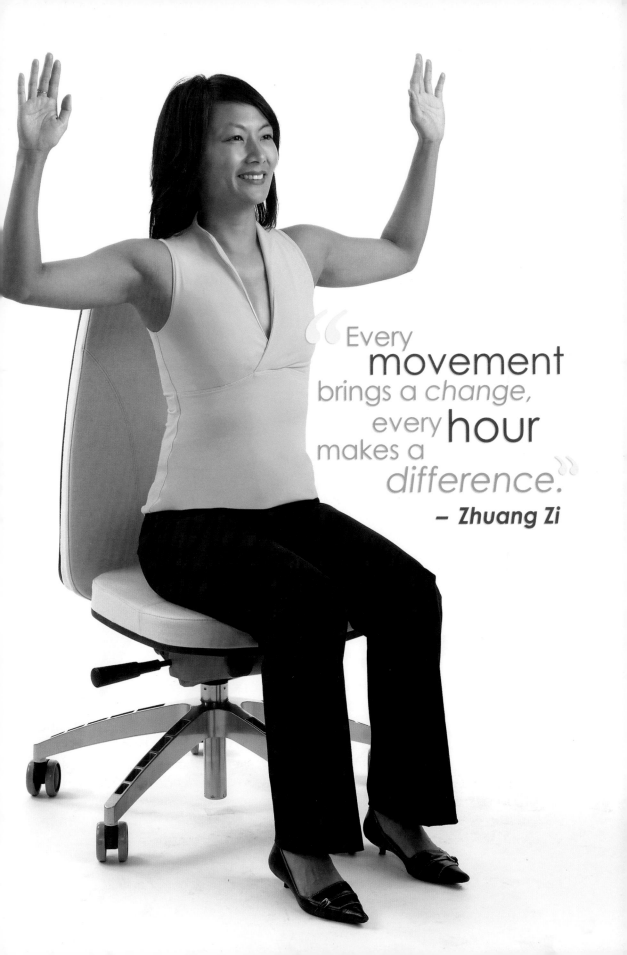

"Every **movement** brings a *change*, every **hour** makes a *difference*."

— Zhuang Zi

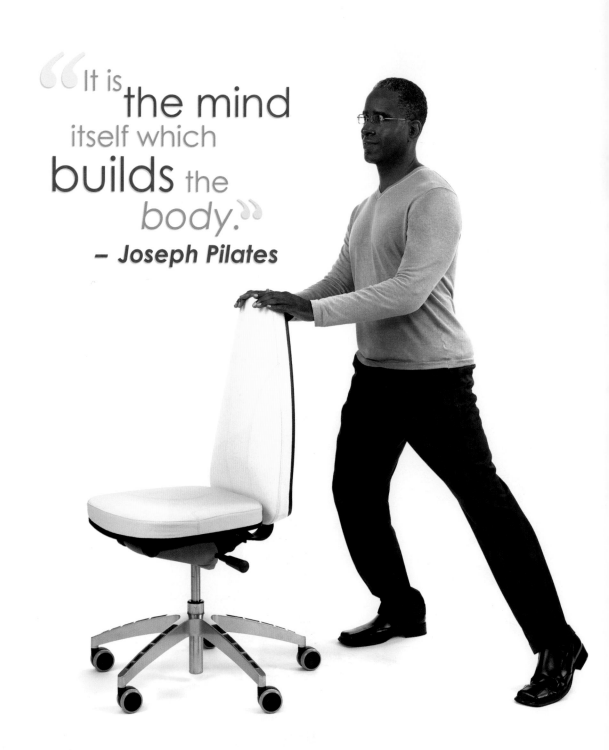

"It is the mind itself which builds the body."

— Joseph Pilates

Contents

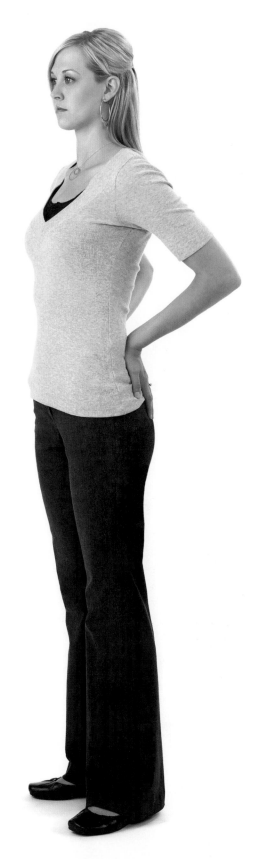

"Physical fitness is the first requisite to happiness."

— Joseph Pilates

Inviting Pilates into Your Day

Do you remember recess?

Recess was that wonderful time when you stopped the important tasks you were doing to go out and play. You let your mind take a break from spelling lists and multiplication tables, and you moved and stretched your muscles in every possible way—jumping, rolling, and even hanging upside down. You laughed out loud and deeply breathed the fresh air, rejuvenating your body and recharging your brain.

The majority of us are now missing these essential components of recess. We have become increasingly sedentary in our work, home, and leisure activities, to the point that we no longer explore the full motion of our spines, hips, or shoulders. Many of us have become removed from seeing, feeling, or knowing joyful, centered movement. Stress, prolonged sitting and standing, awkward positioning, and repetitive activities have negatively affected our posture, our movements, and our strength.

Do you find yourself slouched forward over your desk, straining your back and tensing your neck, with your shoulders scrunched up to your ears? Do you get so engrossed in a project that you suddenly realize your body is stiff and sore from being in the same position too long? How often do you listen to your body's needs?

As an occupational therapist, my introduction to Pilates initially focused on its methods and movements as rehabilitation tools, helping people with pain and limited strength or mobility, to regain function. I soon realized that Pilates exercises effectively improve core stability and body mobility, with the vital added benefit of encouraging people to truly become aware of how they use and misuse their bodies. This awareness is beneficial for clients recovering from injury or illness, as well as for the millions of us who sit too much each day.

Like the balanced, joyful movement of the child on the playground, Pilates exercise helps to reconnect your body to your brain, deepen your breathing patterns, improve your confidence with movement, strengthen your body from the inside out, increase the variety of your movements, and decrease your muscle tension. Our bodies are designed for movement, and Pilates provides effective guidelines for exercise, as well as for using healthy positions and movements in our everyday activities.

Desk Pilates is an invitation to bring the benefits of a little recess into each day—to be mindful of your breathing, to explore body-mind connections, to effectively utilize core muscles to support your spine, to increase your awareness of posture and positioning, and to playfully emphasize strength and flexibility throughout your daily activities—even while sitting at your desk!

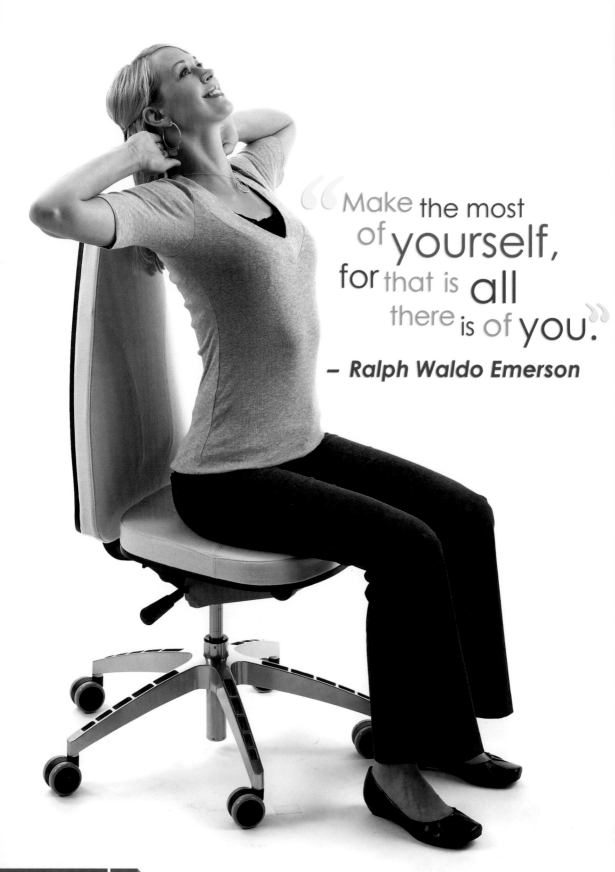

" Make the most of yourself, for that is all there is of you."

– Ralph Waldo Emerson

Introducing Pilates

Desk Pilates is different from many other forms of exercise because it invites you to move mindfully, focus on your breathing, and strengthen your deep postural muscles. The exercises have been adapted so that no special equipment is required, and the movements can be done anytime, right in your chair at work, at home, or anywhere. Every person can benefit from Pilates, whether young or old, athletic or sedentary.

As you get started, keep these guidelines in mind—

> Listen to your body and your own capabilities; choose only the movements that feel comfortable. Never force any movement or try to go beyond your limit.
> Progress gradually; build on your successes.
> Perform standing exercises close to your desk, with fingertips on a firm surface if needed for balance.
> Consult with your health care provider before beginning any fitness program, especially if you have health concerns.
> Stop and rest if, during any exercise, you experience discomfort or feel light-headed.

This book introduces you to Pilates principles and to your body's core muscles, then gives a practical exploration of Pilates fundamentals that align your body while sitting. The *Desk Pilates* exercise sequence can be performed in its entirety, or you can start benefiting by including just a few mind-body movements at various times during your day. Choose Pilates exercises that encourage motion in ways other than how your body routinely moves—like bending backward or sideways.

For overall health, Pilates exercise should be supplemented most days of the week by aerobic exercise such as brisk walking, for a total of at least thirty minutes—five or ten minute segments do add up. Applying Pilates fundamentals to walking and other forms of exercise will additionally enhance your safe, effective performance, and help prevent injury.

Remember that water is also essential for your optimal body and brain function, and is best absorbed by drinking small amounts frequently during the day. Reflecting on this theme, include water as well as Pilates often in your everyday routine, and fuel your body and mind with good nutrition.

Desk Pilates provides many of the basics you would find in a beginning Pilates class, but it is not meant to substitute for individual or group sessions with a qualified instructor who can address your body's unique needs. As you explore incorporating Pilates principles and movements into your day and experience some of the benefits, you will very likely be interested in learning more. Pilates resources, including how to find an instructor, are listed on page 46.

Every person can benefit from Pilates, whether young or old, athletic or sedentary.

Learning Pilates

Pilates has been called the ultimate mind-body exercise system, a whole approach to movement emphasizing body alignment, breathing, strength, flexibility, balance, and endurance. Joseph Pilates (1880-1967) formulated his ideas from his study of yoga, meditation, gymnastics, martial arts, weight training and calisthenics. Contemporary Pilates continues to build on his original principles and teachings, while also incorporating current exercise science and knowledge about the human body.

More than just a series of exercises, Pilates provides a method of achieving intelligent fitness for lifelong health. The holistic emphasis teaches consciousness and care during movement, including throughout the performance of our daily self-care, work, and play activities. Pilates is a mind-body lifestyle that is embodied in how we choose to sit and stand and breathe, and how we choose to approach everyday life.

In addition to enhancing physical fitness and overall enjoyment of life, Joseph Pilates' writings identified several concepts that underlie the meaning and effectiveness of his whole body exercise system. Learning Pilates is an evolving process, and consistent practice is important for positive outcomes. By including Pilates principles and movements within your everyday life, even your routine tasks become opportunities to practice the techniques, inviting mindfulness to whatever you are doing and experiencing—whether talking on the phone, writing at your desk, or sitting at your computer.

Pilates provides a method of achieving intelligent fitness for lifelong health.

Key Pilates principles include –

CONCENTRATION — Pilates exercise targets both mental and physical training, requiring continual awareness of how your body is moving. Your focused attention keeps you in the present moment, deepening your understanding, as well as increasing the benefits of the movement.

ALIGNMENT — Attending to proper alignment of the body during sitting and standing positions allows safe, effective use of muscles in balanced ways.

CONTROL — The beginning and ending of each movement is consciously controlled, as is the transition from one movement to another.

CENTERING — Each movement initiates from your body's center, the core muscles that support the spine. From your strong center, the body moves in three planes—forward and backward, rotating, and bending sideways.

PRECISION — Movement precision allows detailed focus on the muscles needed for a particular movement, while relaxing other muscles, encouraging whole body integration.

BREATH — Breathing is coordinated with each movement. Proper breathing provides increased lung capacity, calms the mind and body, and activates targeted muscles.

FLUIDITY — Dynamic, graceful movement flows when muscles are used in specific sequences, performed smoothly and evenly.

Connecting with Your Core

The Pilates method emphasizes the concept of a strong center that provides the core stability your body needs to support your spine during daily activities as well as exercise. The body's core is three-dimensional, with muscles spanning from the rib cage to the pelvis, the low back, and hips. Connecting with your core muscles will maximize your benefits from Pilates.

Core muscles include deep muscles such as transversus abdominis, lumbar multifidus, pelvic floor, and diaphragm, as well as outer layers of muscles—internal and external obliques, rectus abdominis, quadratus lumborum, erector spinae, and gluteals. Your inner core muscles brace and support your lower spine, while outer core muscles move your trunk—bending your spine forward and backward, rotating, and bending from side to side.

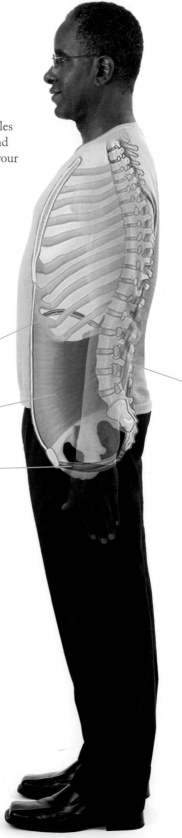

diaphragm

transversus abdominis

pelvic floor

multifidus

Thinking about and activating the muscles of your inner core (labeled above) provides the essential stability for your spine during Pilates, as well as other activities. Try visualizing your inner core as a cylinder, with transversus abdominis in the front and sides, multifidus in back, the diaphragm at the top of the cylinder, and the pelvic floor muscles at the bottom.

Pilates exercises encourage subtle (less than 25% of maximum) contraction of transversus abdominis, with the sensation of gently bracing. These muscle fibers wrap horizontally from front to back like a corset, and they can best be felt at the bikini line when drawing your lower abdomen toward the spine.

Multifidus, which connects the vertebral segments of your low back, works together with transversus abdominis to support your inner core.

When you breathe deeply and exhale fully, the dome-shaped diaphragm lowers and lifts in your abdomen, facilitating the contraction of your deep inner core muscles.

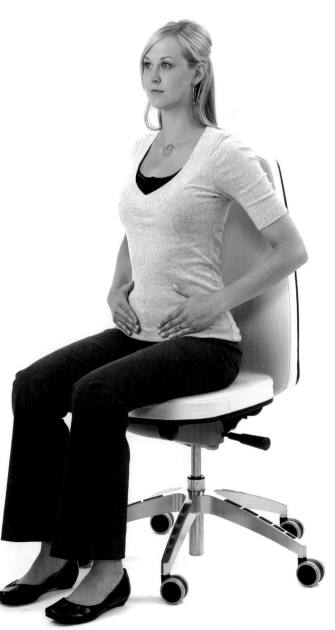

Contracting the pelvic floor muscles (Kegel exercise) also helps to activate transversus abdominis. Think of the pelvic floor as a diamond-shaped muscular hammock at the bottom of the pelvic opening, spanning the area from the pubic bone in the front, the left and right sit bones, and the tailbone in back. Imagine gently bringing the four points together without clenching, then lifting that center point up like an elevator in the lower abdomen. It is important to also relax the pelvic floor muscles.

Inhale, and as you exhale, gently lift the pelvic floor—as if walking into cold water, and then activate transversus abdominis, flattening the abdomen by gently tightening—like zipping up a tight pair of jeans from your pubic bone to your belly button.

With practice, this sensation of inner core support will become habit, providing the stability your trunk needs prior to moving your arms or legs during walking, exercise, and daily activities. *Desk Pilates* exercises activate both the deep core muscles that stabilize and the outer layers of muscles that mobilize—effectively strengthening your body from the inside out.

Moving in Three Dimensions

Our bodies are designed for movement—every day, in all directions. Pilates targets a strong center, with a spine that moves freely and with control in all three planes of motion. The inner core braces and supports, while outer core muscles move your trunk.

Internal and external obliques, together with rectus abdominis, bend your spine forward. Abdominals stabilize while erector spinae and multifidus bend your spine backward.

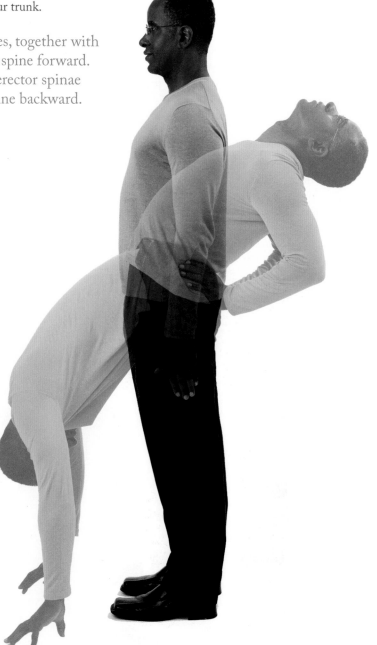

Internal and external obliques activate with quadratus lumborum, multifidus, and erector spinae for side bending, and obliques work together with erector spinae for trunk rotation. Deeper spinal muscles also activate, assisting segmental motion of the spine while bending backward, side bending, and rotating.

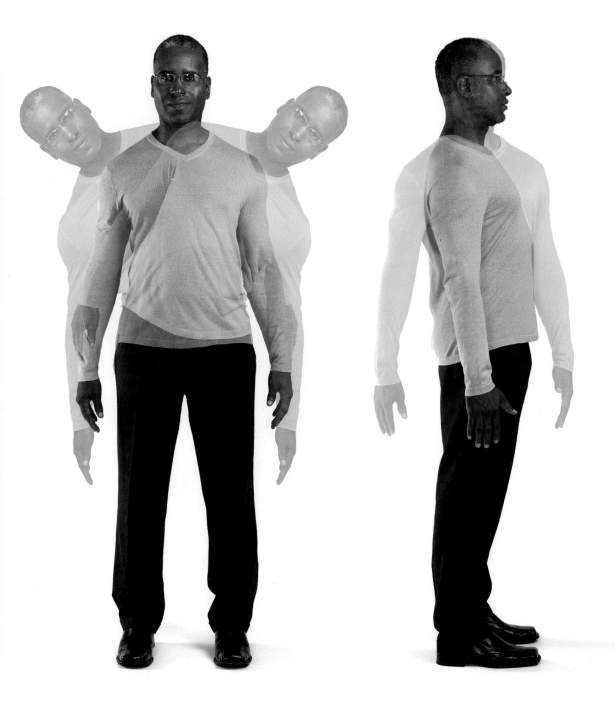

Exploring Pilates Basics

Pilates fundamentals encourage awareness and appreciation of your body and how it moves, and can be applied to any exercise or activity. The basic principles of breathing and optimal placement of the pelvis, rib cage, shoulders, head and neck all work together for safe, effective, controlled movement.

To explore Pilates exercise while sitting, begin by sitting tall, evenly on your sit bones in the center of a sturdy chair, allowing enough space for your arms and legs to move. Place your feet comfortably on the floor (or if needed, on a small footrest or a book) a few inches apart, with toes pointed forward. Your thighs should be parallel (or slightly sloping downward) to the floor, and legs parallel with one another. Keep your knees centered over your ankles, and in line with the second toe of each foot.

Proper alignment of your body during sitting and standing allows comfortable, efficient use of muscles in balanced ways. Your postural alignment simply refers to the position of your body in space. Although there is no "perfect" posture, an "ideal" posture keeps the stresses on the body evenly distributed so your joints are bearing weight comfortably and muscles are working optimally. Ideal posture is not rigid and tense, but is lengthened and aligned.

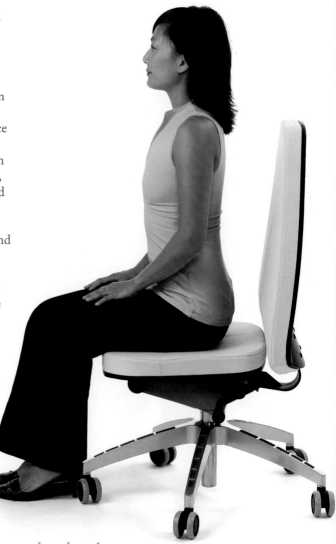

Your body position is very important during Pilates exercise, and most often you will start and end each movement with neutral spine alignment. An ideally aligned, neutral spine runs down the center of your body, and from the side it displays three natural curves. Your pelvis provides the foundation for your spine, with gentle "C" curves behind your lower back and neck, and a backward "C" curve at your upper middle back.

Breathing

If you were to include only one Pilates principle within your daily life, awareness of your breathing would have the greatest impact. Attention to your breath is an essential exercise in and of itself. A full, relaxed breath pattern effectively oxygenates your body, calms your neuromuscular system, and focuses your mind.

Breathing is coordinated with each movement to help engage core muscles and release unnecessary tension, allowing you to focus on each moment. Because the most efficient exchange of gases occurs in the lower lobes of the lungs, try a full natural breath pattern—exhaling completely to empty your lungs, breathing in through the nose and out through the mouth.

Place your hands gently on your outer ribs.

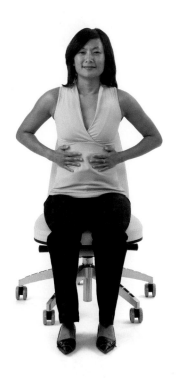

Inhale, through your nose
Feel your breath expanding wide into the sides and the back of your rib cage, and your hands moving slightly away from one another.

Focus on exhaling completely, feel abdominal engagement, then allow your next breath to be full and natural. Release your pelvic floor muscles as you inhale, while maintaining subtle (less than 25% of maximum) contraction of your transversus abdominis.

Exhale, through your mouth
Slowly and gently lift your pelvic floor and tighten deep abdominal muscles, and feel the ribs releasing in toward the center of your body, with your hands moving closer together again.

Pelvis

Awareness of the optimal position of your pelvis and the feeling of abdominal connection are vital at the start of every Pilates exercise. Neutral pelvis is typically defined when the top front pelvic bones and the pubic bone are in the same plane, honoring the natural curve of your low back.

To check, place the heels of your hands at the bony prominences at the tops of the front of each pelvic bone and angle your fingertips down toward the pubic bone, making a triangle that is vertical when standing or sitting, and horizontal when lying down. These bony prominences at the tops of the front of your pelvis will also be relatively level with those at the tops of the back of your pelvis.

Balance your pelvis by rocking forward and back, exploring the movement of your lumbar spine.

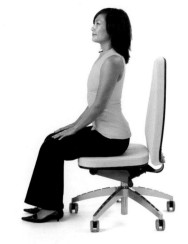

Inhale
Rock your pelvis forward, increasing the arch of your lower back.

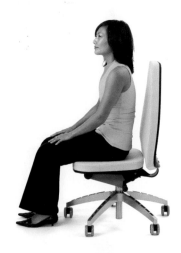

Exhale
Contract abdominals and rock your pelvis backward, flattening and then gently bending your low back.

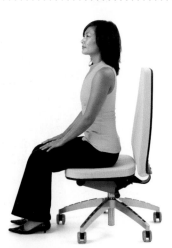

Repeat this a few times, and then find the center where your pelvis is neutral, sitting tall on your sit bones and maintaining the natural "C" curve of your low back.

Rib Cage

Maintain abdominal engagement to keep your rib cage in good alignment directly over your pelvis when sitting and standing, and when moving your arms. Emphasize breathing into the sides and back of your rib cage, focusing on keeping your abdominal connection during inhalation, and enhancing the connection during exhalation.

Balance your rib cage over your pelvis by allowing it to move gently forward and back.

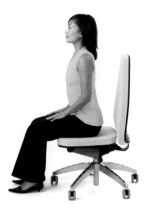

Inhale
Expand the rib cage, pressing your shoulders back.

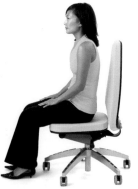

Exhale
Reverse the motion, as though caving in your chest.

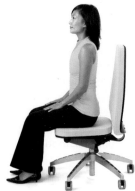

Then find center, where your ribs are directly over your hips.

Explore the abdominal connection from your rib cage to your pelvis, adding arm movement. Start with your arms long by your sides, palms facing one another.

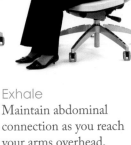

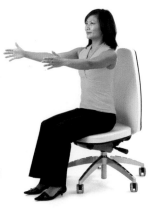

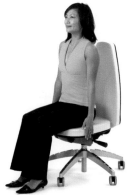

Inhale
Raise your arms to shoulder height.

Exhale
Maintain abdominal connection as you reach your arms overhead, keeping your rib cage directly over your pelvis without allowing your ribs to move forward.

Inhale
Lower your arms to the front of your shoulders again.

Exhale
Maintain abdominal engagement and lower your arms down by your sides.

Shoulder Blades

Position your shoulder blades flat against your rib cage, with a feeling of gliding along the rib cage during movement. Maintain a sensation of openness and width across the front and back of your shoulders, without allowing the shoulders to round forward or the shoulder blades to overly squeeze back. At the start of every Pilates exercise, be aware of stabilizing your shoulder blades against the rib cage, gently sliding them back and down toward your spine as in a "V".

Sit with neutral pelvis and spine, your arms reaching in front of your shoulders, with palms facing one another, and your elbows softly straight.

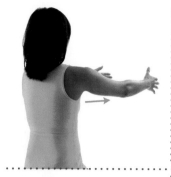

Inhale
Reach your fingertips forward, allowing your shoulder blades to glide around the rib cage as they move away from your spine.

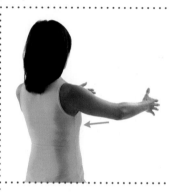

Exhale
Gently squeeze your shoulder blades back and down toward your spine.

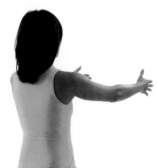

After exploring the end ranges, find the middle of this movement, with your shoulder blades in neutral position, flat against your rib cage.

Allow your arms to relax comfortably by your sides.

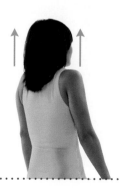

Inhale
Gently shrug your shoulders up toward your ears.

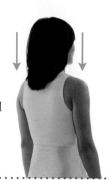

Exhale
Slide the shoulder blades back and down, finding neutral position, flat against the rib cage.

Head and Neck

Keep the natural "C" curve of your neck, with your head centered and directly above your shoulders. This is especially important since many of our routine daily activities unfortunately encourage a forward-head posture. During Pilates movements, your neck will typically continue the line created by the rest of your spine when bending your spine forward, extending backward, bending sideways or rotating.

From the side view while standing or sitting, optimally your ears are in line over your shoulders, over your rib cage, over your hips. This relaxed, aligned posture gives a feeling of lengthening through your spine, as though a string were attached to the top of your head, gently pulling up to elongate your spine.

Sit with your pelvis and spine neutral, legs parallel, feet hip-distance apart. Shoulders are relaxed, abdominals engaged.

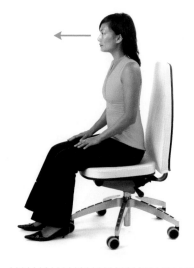

Inhale
Allow your head to move slowly forward, keeping your head level.

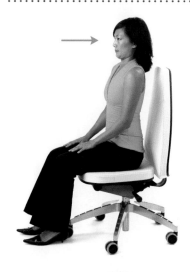

Exhale
Gently glide your head slowly and steadily straight backward, keeping your head level and your eyes looking forward.

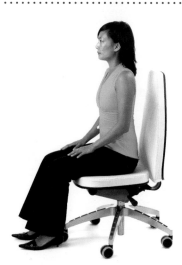

Balance your head and neck, feeling the movement backward and forward. After exploring the end ranges, find the middle of this movement, where your neck is neutral with its natural curve, and the muscles in front and back of your neck feel relaxed.

Aligning While Sitting

How many hours do you actually spend sitting each day—including driving, commuting, eating, working, reading, using a computer, attending concerts or sports events, socializing, or watching movies or television?

When sitting, your spine experiences nearly twice the stress as when you are standing, and slouching while sitting increases the pressure even more. Optimal posture during sitting focuses on neutral alignment of your spine, honoring the three natural curves at the neck, middle back and lower back.

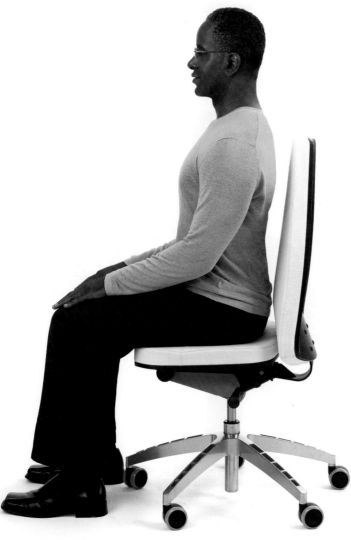

Special considerations during sitting:

> Head and eyes level
> Neck neutral and tension free
> Chin parallel to floor
> Shoulders relaxed
> Chest broad and slightly lifted
> Elbows slightly open at sides
> Neutral pelvis
> Lengthened spine, natural curves
> Feet comfortably on floor or footrest
> Flat abdomen
> Lumbar curve, support if needed
> Thighs supported, parallel to floor or slightly sloping downward
> Buttocks to the back of chair
> Sitting evenly on sit bones
> Wrists neutral, hands relaxed
> Maintain your strong center

Exercising
with Desk Pilates

Desk Pilates exercises invite greater body awareness and opportunities for frequent, varied movement throughout your day. You can perform the entire sequence or mix portions into each day, a few minutes every hour to keep your body and your mind in balance. Remember to choose exercises that move your body in ways that are not typical within your routine daily activities—such as bending your spine backward or sideways.

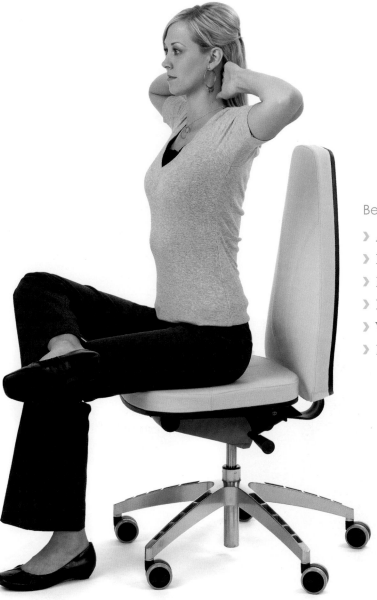

Be mindful to —

❯ Align your spine in neutral

❯ Breathe deeply, exhaling fully

❯ Engage abdominals

❯ Lengthen through your spine

❯ Widen across your chest

❯ Relax neck and shoulders

Spine Lengthening

Repeat 3-5 times

Start
Sit tall, neutral pelvis and spine, abdominals engaged, with feet flat and hip-width apart.

Inhale
Expand breath into the sides and back of your rib cage.

Exhale
Lift your pelvic floor muscles and tighten your abdominals, elongate through your entire spine, gently lift your sternum, widening across your chest, allowing your shoulder blades to drop back and down.

› Listen to your body, performing only movement that feels comfortable.

› Tighten your abdominals, supporting your spine throughout movement.

› Stay wide across the front of your shoulders and collarbones.

› Keep your shoulder blades sliding back and down, and your neck relaxed.

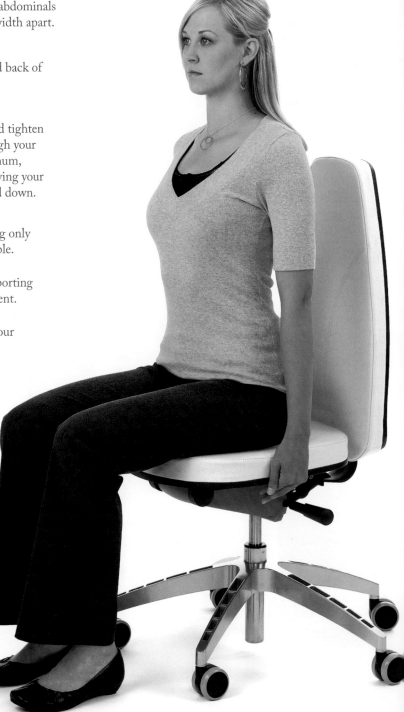

Hundred

Continue for 100 counts with slow
5 count breaths

Start
Sit tall, neutral pelvis and spine,
abdominals engaged, with feet flat and
hip-width apart, your arms long by
your sides, with palms facing forward
(variations include palms facing
backward or facing your body).

Inhale for 5 counts
Lengthen through your spine, pulsing
your arms back from the shoulders with
each count, as though you are pressing
on springs with the back of your hands.

Exhale for 5 counts
Tighten your abdominals, continuing
to rhythmically pulse your arms back
for each count.

> Listen to your body, performing
  only movement that feels
  comfortable.

> Maintain abdominal connection,
  stabilizing your spine
  throughout the movement.

> Pumping motion comes from
  your shoulder joints, while
  staying wide across the front
  and back of shoulders.

> Stabilize your shoulder blades
  and rib cage throughout,
  avoiding upper body tension.

> Keep your eyes gazing forward,
  your neck aligned and relaxed.

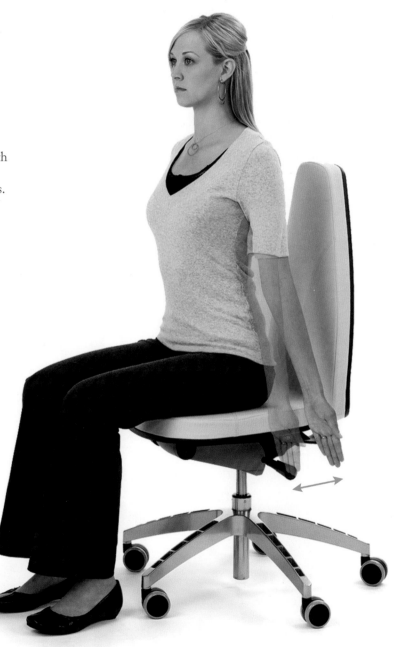

Neck
Turn

Repeat 3 times, alternating directions

Start
Sit tall, neutral pelvis and spine, abdominals engaged, with feet flat and hip-width apart.

Inhale
Lengthen through your spine, ensuring neutral neck position, with your head and eyes level.

Exhale
Tighten your abdominals, and gently rotate your neck to look over one shoulder, keeping your head level.

Inhale
Maintain the rotated neck position, with your shoulders relaxed.

Exhale
Keeping abdominal connection, slowly return your neck to center.

❭ Listen to your body, performing only movement that feels comfortable.

❭ Maintain abdominal connection, supporting your spine throughout the movement.

❭ Stay wide across the front of your shoulders and collarbones.

❭ Keep your shoulder blades sliding back and down.

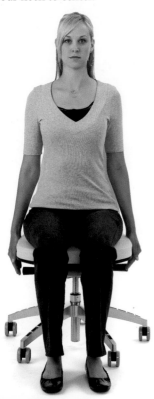 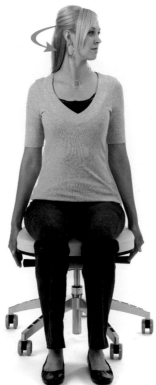 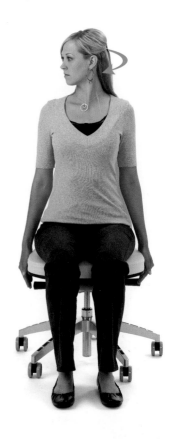

Neck
Side Bend

Repeat 3 times, alternating directions

Start
Sit tall, neutral pelvis and spine, abdominals engaged, with feet flat and hip-width apart.

Inhale
Lengthen through your spine, ensuring neutral neck position, with head and eyes level.

Exhale
Tighten your abdominals, and gently lengthen your neck up and over sideways, allowing your ear to move closer to your shoulder.

Inhale
Maintain side bend position, with your shoulders relaxed.

Exhale
Keep abdominal connection, and slowly lengthen your neck and return to center.

❭ Listen to your body, performing only movement that feels comfortable.

❭ Maintain abdominal connection, supporting your spine throughout movement.

❭ Stay wide across the front of your shoulders and collarbones.

❭ Keep your shoulder blades sliding back and down.

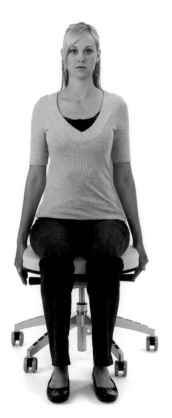
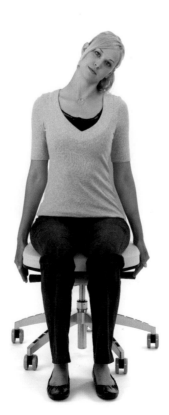
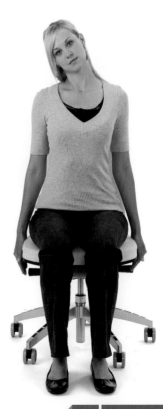

Shoulder Reach

Repeat 5-8 times

Start

Sit tall, neutral pelvis and spine, abdominals engaged, with feet flat and hip-width apart. With your arms long and lifted to shoulder height, interlace your fingers with palms facing away from body.

Inhale

Keep lengthening through your spine and gently press your arms forward. Your shoulder blades glide around the rib cage while moving away from your spine.

Exhale

Tighten your abdominals, then slide your shoulder blades back and down toward your spine in a "V", widening across the front and back of your shoulders. Feel your shoulder blades stabilized flat against the rib cage

❯ Listen to your body, performing only movement that feels comfortable.

❯ Maintain abdominal connection, stabilizing your spine throughout movement.

❯ Stay wide across the front of your shoulders and collarbones.

❯ Release your shoulder blades back and down, keeping your neck relaxed

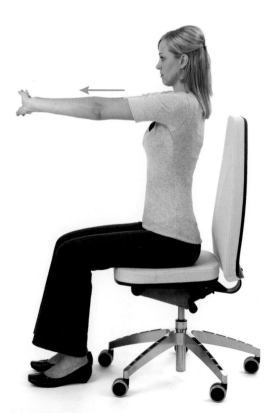 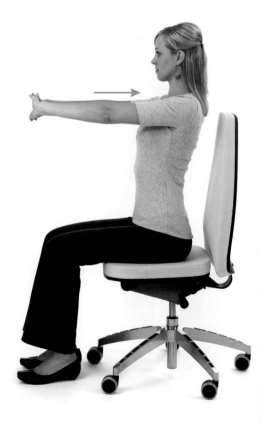

Arm Circles

Repeat 5 times each direction

Start
Sit tall, neutral pelvis and spine, abdominals engaged, with feet flat and hip-width apart, your arms long with palms facing your body.

Inhale
Maintain abdominal connection as you lift your arms overhead, but only as far as rib cage stays aligned directly over pelvis.

Exhale
Tighten abdominals, then circle arms out to your sides and around back down to your hips.

❯ Listen to your body, performing only movement that feels comfortable.

❯ Maintain abdominal connection, stabilizing your spine throughout movement.

❯ Stay wide across the front of the shoulders and collarbones.

❯ Keep your shoulder blades sliding back and down, and your neck relaxed.

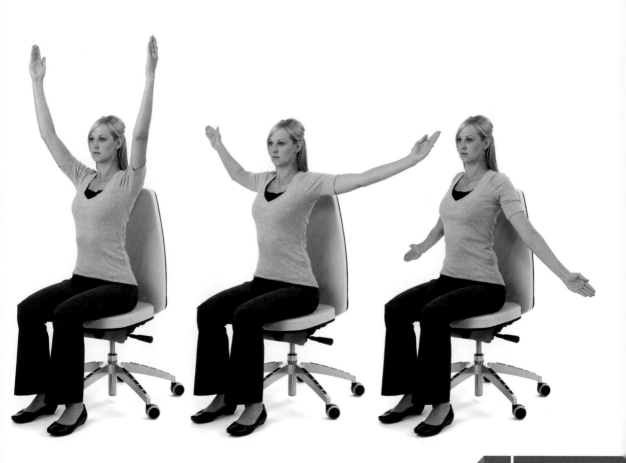

Open
Elbows

Repeat 5-8 times

Start
Sit tall, neutral pelvis and spine, abdominals engaged, with feet flat and hip-width apart. Bend your elbows to 90 degrees at (or slightly below) shoulder height, palms facing one another, open across your chest, your shoulder blades stabilized.

Inhale
Lengthen through your spine.

Exhale
Tighten your abdominals, slowly open your arms out to your sides, palms facing front, expand your chest and slide your shoulder blades back and down.

Inhale
Slowly return your arms to the start position.

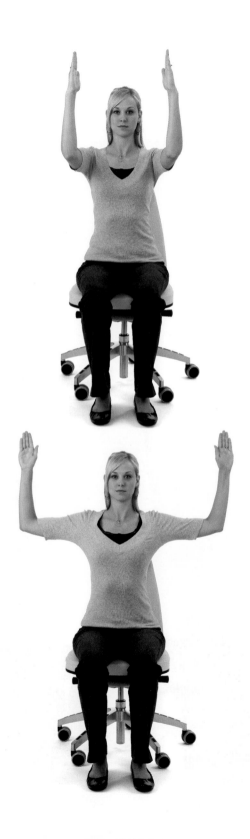

> Listen to your body, performing only movement that feels comfortable.

> Maintain abdominal connection, stabilizing your spine throughout movement.

> Stay wide across the front of your shoulders and collarbones.

> Keep your shoulder blades sliding back and down, and your neck relaxed.

Elbow
Reach

Repeat 5 times alternating sides,
and 5 times together

Start
Sit tall, neutral pelvis and spine, abdominals
engaged, with feet flat and hip-width apart.
Bend elbows 90 degrees at your sides, palms
facing, open across chest, your shoulders relaxed.

Inhale
Lengthen through your spine.

Exhale
Tighten your abdominals and slowly reach your
elbow(s) toward the ceiling with your hand(s)
over your shoulder(s).

Inhale
Keeping your abdominals engaged, slowly
return your arm(s) to the start position.

❯ Listen to your body, performing only
movement that feels comfortable.

❯ Maintain abdominal connection,
stabilizing your spine throughout
movement.

❯ Stay wide across the front of your
shoulders and collarbones.

❯ Keep your shoulder blades sliding back
and down, and your neck relaxed.

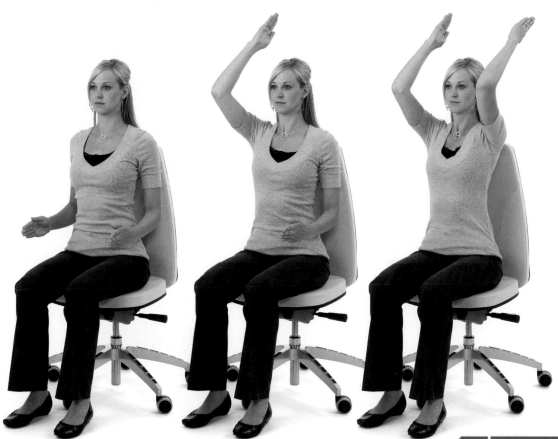

Spine Twist

Repeat 5-8 times, alternating directions

Start

Sit tall, neutral pelvis and spine, abdominals engaged, with feet flat and hip-width apart, your arms long and lifted to shoulder height, palms facing one another, while keeping your shoulder blades stabilized back and down.

Inhale

Lengthen through your spine.

Exhale

Tighten your abdominals, keeping your pelvis stable, then slowly rotate your spine for 3 counts, spiraling tall. Bend your elbow as you rotate to that direction, while reaching the opposite arm forward.

Inhale

Maintain abdominal connection, and return to center start position, staying lengthened through spine.

Exhale

Contract abdominals, keeping your pelvis stable, then slowly rotate your spine the other direction for 3 counts, bending your back elbow.

> Listen to your body, performing only movement that feels comfortable.

> Maintain abdominal connection, supporting your spine throughout movement.

> Keep lengthened through your spine, your shoulder blades sliding back and down.

> Move only as far as feels comfortable in each direction.

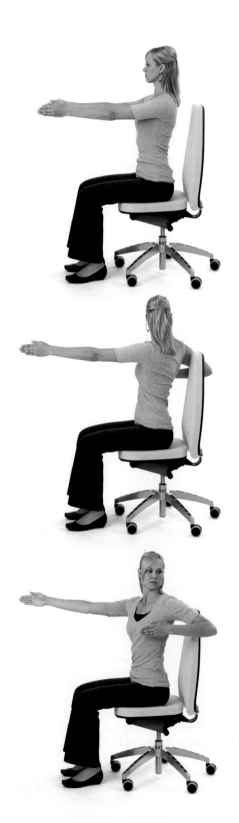

Sternum
Lift

Repeat 5-8 times

Start
Sit tall, neutral pelvis and spine, abdominals engaged, with feet flat and hip-width apart. With your fingertips behind your head (not neck) to support the weight of your head, reach your elbows wide to the sides.

Inhale
Lengthen through your spine.

Exhale
Tighten your abdominals, and slowly extend your neck and upper back backward, looking to the ceiling.

Inhale
Maintain this lifted position, reaching your sternum to the ceiling.

Exhale
With your core strong, slowly return your spine to vertical.

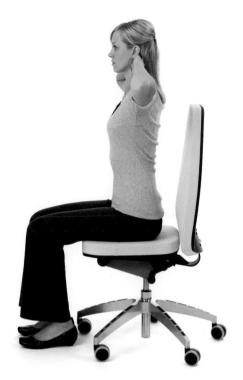

> Listen to your body, performing only movement that feels comfortable.

> Maintain abdominal connection, supporting your spine throughout movement.

> Extend your upper-middle back as far as you feel comfortable and in control.

> Stay wide across the front and back of your shoulders, elbows reaching wide.

> Keep your shoulder blades sliding back and down, and your neck relaxed.

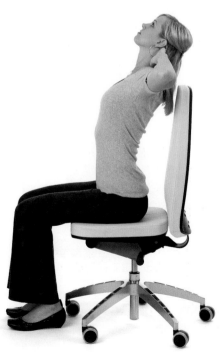

Gluteal Squeeze

Repeat 5-8 times

Start
Sit tall, neutral pelvis and spine, abdominals engaged, with feet flat and hip-width apart your arms alongside body, your shoulder blades stabilized, and your hands on your lap or gently pressing into the sides of your chair.

Inhale
Lengthen through your spine.

Exhale
Lift your pelvic floor and tighten your abdominals, keeping pelvis stable, and slowly contract gluteal muscles, squeezing buttocks, slightly lifting off the chair.

Inhale
Maintaining abdominal connection, relax your gluteals and pelvic floor muscles.

❯ Listen to your body, performing only movement that feels comfortable.

❯ Maintain abdominal connection, stabilizing your spine throughout movement.

❯ Keep lengthened through your spine, with shoulder blades sliding back and down.

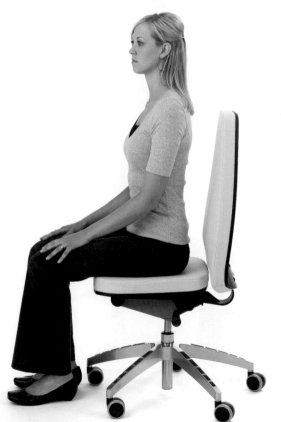
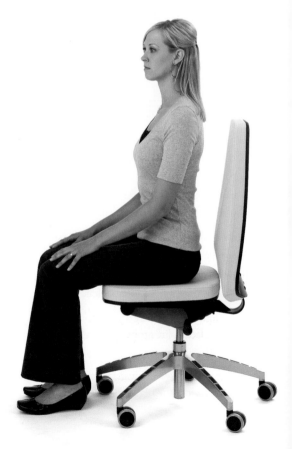

Knee
Drop

Repeat 5-8 times, alternating sides

Start
Sit tall at the front edge of your chair, neutral pelvis and spine, abdominals engaged, your feet flat and hip-width apart, with your arms alongside your body, your shoulder blades stabilized, and your hands gently pressing into the sides of the chair.

Inhale
Lengthen through your spine.

Exhale
Tighten your abdominals, keeping your pelvis stable, and slowly rotate one hip, dropping your knee out to the side, allowing your foot to move along with your leg.

Inhale
Maintain knee drop position, abdominals engaged.

Exhale
Contract abdominals, keeping your pelvis stable, and slowly bring your hip and leg back to the start position.

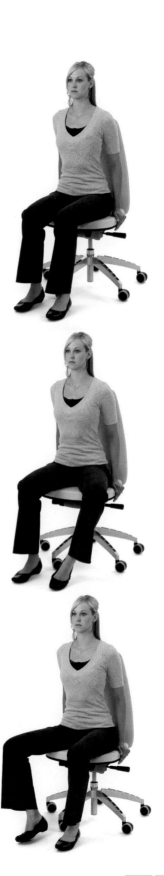

❯ Listen to your body, performing only movement that feels comfortable.

❯ Maintain abdominal connection, stabilizing your spine throughout movement.

❯ Keep lengthened through your spine, with your shoulder blades sliding back and down.

❯ Initiate leg movement from your hip, rotating your leg while your pelvis remains stable.

Leg
Lift

Repeat 5-8 times on one side,
then the other

Start

Sit tall at the front edge of your chair, with
neutral pelvis and spine, abdominals engaged, and
legs at hip-width apart, one knee bent with the
foot flat, the other leg extended and rotated out
from your hip. With your arms alongside your
body and your shoulder blades stabilized, gently
press your hands into the sides of the chair.

Inhale

Lengthen through your spine, contract the
thigh muscles of your extended leg, sliding
your kneecap.

Exhale

Tighten your abdominals, keeping your pelvis
stable, and slowly lift your long leg from the hip,
raising your inner thigh toward the ceiling.

Inhale

Maintain the leg lift position with your
abdominals engaged.

Exhale

Contract your abdominals, keeping your pelvis
stable, then slowly bring your leg back to the start
position, staying turned out from the hip.

> Listen to your body, performing only
> movement that feels comfortable.

> Maintain abdominal connection, stabilizing
> your spine throughout movement.

> Keep lengthened through your spine, with your
> shoulder blades sliding back and down.

> Initiate leg movement from your hip, lifting
> your leg while your pelvis remains stable.

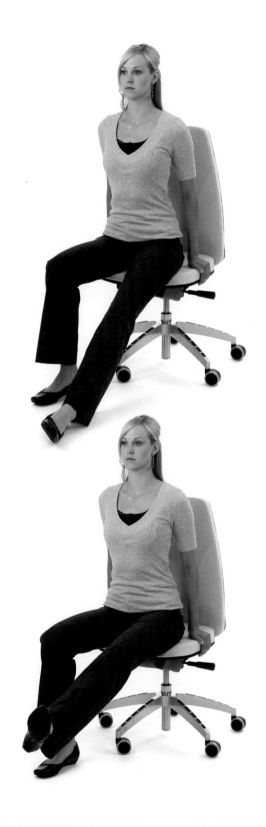

Hip
Hinge

Repeat 5-8 times on one side,
then the other

Start

Sit tall with neutral pelvis and spine,
abdominals engaged, hip of one leg rotated
out with ankle crossed over opposite knee
and hands gently behind your head, your
arms bent, with your elbows reaching wide.

Inhale

Lengthen through your spine, allowing the
hip of your lifted leg to open out to the side
as far as feels comfortable.

Exhale

Tighten your abdominals, then hinge
forward from your hips, keeping your spine
neutral and sternum lifted.

Inhale

Maintain forward hinged position.

Exhale

Contract abdominals, and return to vertical
sitting position.

> Listen to your body, performing only
> movement that feels comfortable.

> Maintain abdominal connection,
> stabilizing your spine throughout
> movement.

> Keep lengthened through your
> spine while hinging forward, as
> though reaching up and out of your
> pelvis.

> Keep both sit bones in contact with
> your chair, with the hip of the lifted
> leg opened out to one side.

> Stay wide across the front and
> back of your shoulders, with your
> sternum lifted.

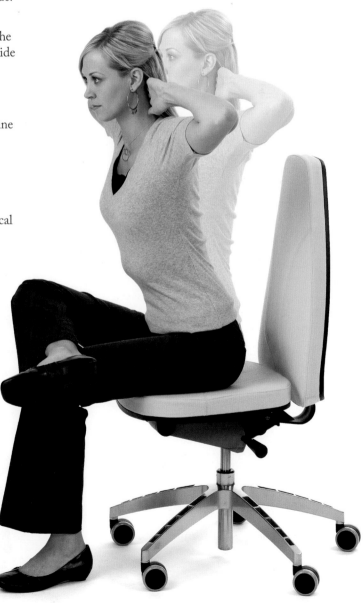

Spine
Stretch Forward

Repeat 5-8 times

Start
Sit tall with neutral pelvis and spine, abdominals engaged, hands resting on your legs that are slightly wider than shoulder-width apart, with your feet flat.

Inhale
Lengthen through your spine.

Exhale
Tighten your abdominals, gently nod your head forward, then slowly and sequentially curve your spine forward, keeping your pelvis vertical, allowing your arms to reach forward.

Inhale
Maintain a curved position, breathing into the sides and back of your rib cage.

Exhale
Contract abdominals to stack your spine up vertically, from bottom to top, returning to tall sitting.

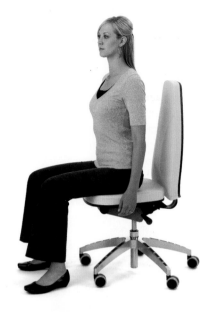

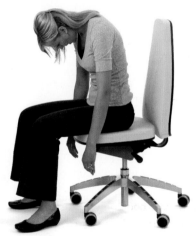

> Avoid this exercise if you have specific spine issues.

> Listen to your body, performing only movement that feels comfortable.

> Maintain abdominal connection, supporting your spine throughout movement.

> Slowly articulate through your spine, rolling down and rolling up.

> Keep your pelvis vertical, with your shoulder blades sliding back and down.

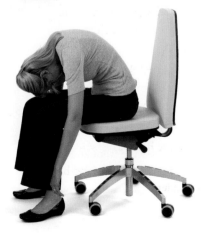

Mermaid

Repeat 3-5 times, alternating sides

Start
Sitting tall, neutral pelvis and spine, abdominals engaged, feet flat at hip-width apart. Hands are resting at sides of chair or your outer thighs.

Inhale
Lengthen through your spine, reaching one arm overhead, gently pressing your other hand into the side of chair or your outer thigh.

Exhale
Tighten abdominals, bending sideways from the top of your spine to the bottom, keeping pelvis level.

Inhale
Return your spine to vertical from bottom to top, again reaching arm overhead.

Exhale
Keep your center strong, lower arm alongside your body.

> Listen to your body, only performing movement that feels comfortable.

> Maintain abdominal connection, supporting spine throughout movement.

> Keep lengthened through your spine while side bending, as though reaching up and out of your pelvis.

> Keep pelvis vertical and level, resisting with opposite hip during side bending.

> Stay wide across the front and back of your shoulders.

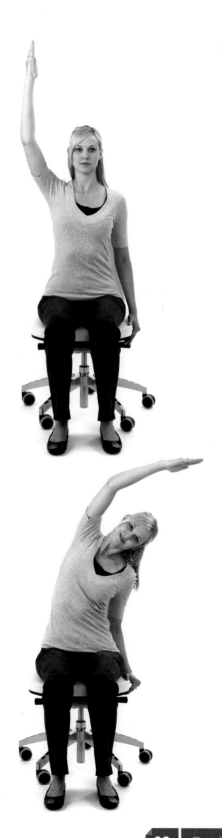

Standing Criss-Cross

Repeat 5-8 times, alternating sides

Start
Stand with neutral pelvis and spine, head level, abdominals engaged, feet parallel at hip-width apart. Shoulders relaxed, and fingertips on firm surface, if needed for balance.

Inhale
Expand breath into sides and back of ribcage, and lengthen through your spine.

Exhale
Tighten abdominals, and lift your left knee, keeping pelvis level. Simultaneously, rotate upper torso toward left, reaching your right arm across body to touch forearm to outside of left knee, staying open across your chest.

Inhale
Slowly return to start position.

Exhale
Contract abdominals, lift your right knee, and rotate upper torso to right.

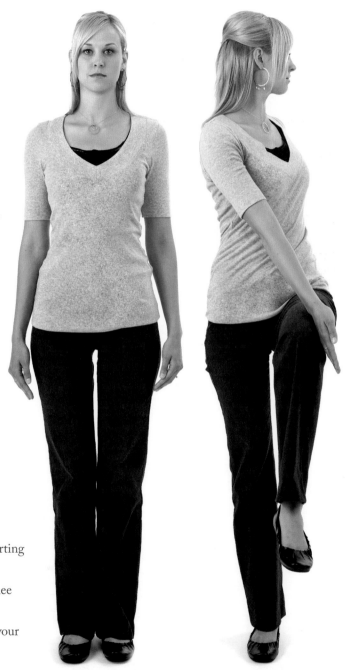

❭ Listen to your body, only performing movement that feels comfortable.

❭ Maintain abdominal connection, supporting spine throughout movement.

❭ Keep pelvis level, without shifting as knee lifts and upper body rotates.

❭ Stay wide across the front and back of your shoulders, neck relaxed.

Bend and Stretch

Repeat 5-8 times

Start
Stand with neutral pelvis and spine, head level, abdominals engaged, feet parallel at hip-width apart. Shoulders relaxed, and fingertips on firm surface, if needed for balance.

Inhale
Bend your knees as far as feels comfortable, keeping your spine neutral and knees aligned over center of feet.

Exhale
Tighten abdominals, and slowly straighten your legs.

Inhale
Lift both heels, rolling through your feet, and keeping your inner thigh and abdominal muscles activated.

Exhale
Contract abdominals, and slowly lower heels, keeping knees and ankles parallel.

› Listen to your body, only performing movement that feels comfortable.

› Maintain abdominal connection, stabilizing spine throughout movement.

› Stay wide across the front and back of your shoulders, neck relaxed.

› Maintain alignment of your knees, ankles, and center of feet.

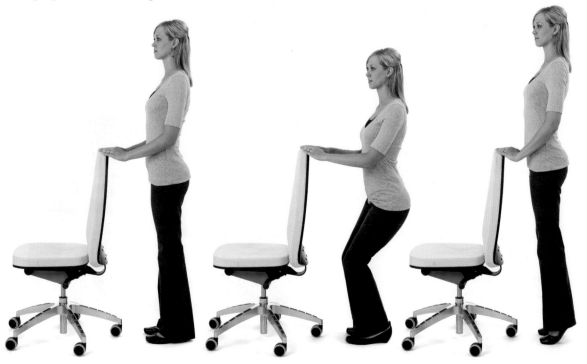

Swimming

Repeat 5-8 times, alternating
sides

Start
Stand with neutral pelvis and spine,
head level, abdominals engaged,
feet parallel at hip-width apart.
Shoulders relaxed, and fingertips on
firm surface, if needed for balance.

Inhale
Expand breath into sides and back
of ribcage, and lengthen through
your spine.

Exhale
Tighten abdominals, lift your right
arm overhead and simultaneously
extend your left leg back, keeping
pelvis level and torso stable.

Inhale
Slowly return to start position.

Exhale
Contract abdominals, lift your left
arm and extend your right leg back.

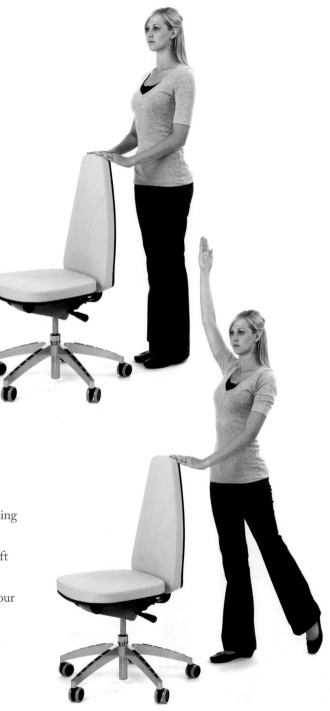

❯ Listen to your body, only performing
movement that feels comfortable.

❯ Maintain abdominal connection, stabilizing
spine throughout movement.

❯ Slide your shoulder blade down as you lift
your arm overhead.

❯ Stay wide across the front and back of your
shoulders, neck relaxed.

❯ Keep torso stable and pelvis level during
opposite arm and leg movements.

Heel Lift
and Lower

Repeat 5-8 times on one side,
then other

Start

Stand with neutral pelvis and spine,
head level, shoulders relaxed, abdominals
engaged, and fingertips on firm surface, if
needed for balance. Bend one knee, and
step the other leg straight back, allowing
your torso to move backward.

Inhale

Bend your back knee and lift your heel,
keeping pelvis and spine neutral.

Exhale

Tighten abdominals, slowly lower heel
toward the floor, lengthening through
your calf.

> Listen to your body, only performing
> movement that feels comfortable.

> Maintain abdominal connection,
> stabilizing spine throughout movement.

> Stay wide across the front and back of
> your shoulders, neck relaxed.

> Maintain stable pelvis, and alignment
> of knees, ankles, and center of feet.

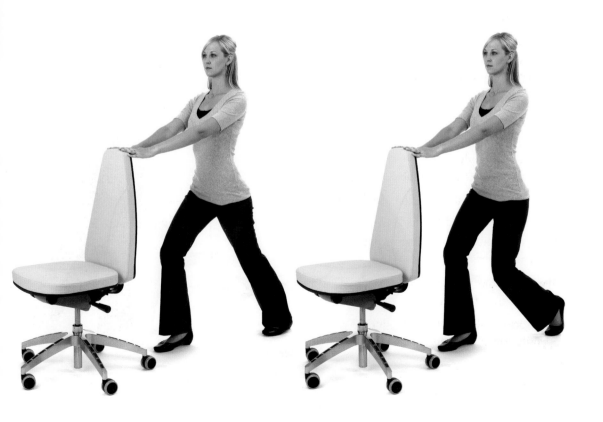

Skating

Repeat 5-8 times, alternating sides

Start
Stand with neutral spine, feet parallel at hip-width apart, abdominals engaged, and fingertips on firm surface, if needed for balance. Slightly bend hips and knees to a comfortable squat position.

Inhale
Keep your pelvis stable and shift your weight to your right leg.

Exhale
Tighten abdominals and slide your left foot out to the side.

Inhale
Return your left leg to start position, and then shift weight onto left leg.

Exhale
Keeping abdominals engaged, slide your right foot out to side.

❯ Listen to your body, only performing movement that feels comfortable.

❯ Maintain abdominal connection, stabilizing spine throughout movement.

❯ Stay wide across the front and back of your shoulders, neck relaxed.

❯ Initiate leg movement from your hip, keeping pelvis stable throughout.

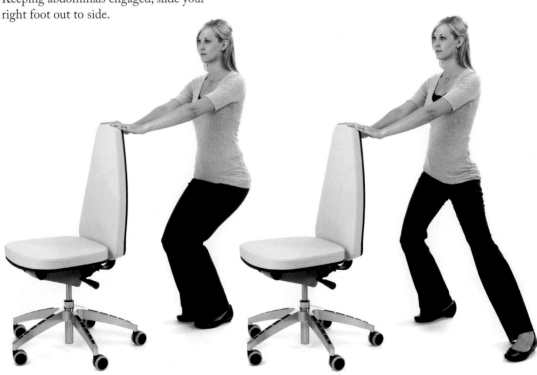

Swan Dive

Repeat 5-8 times

Start
Stand with neutral spine, legs slightly turned out with feet just wider than shoulder-width apart, abdominals engaged, shoulders relaxed, and hands placed at low back for support.

Inhale
Lengthen through your spine, sliding shoulder blades back and down.

Exhale
Tighten abdominals, and slowly arch your spine backward as far as feels comfortable, extending evenly through the spine.

Inhale
Maintain extension of your spine.

Exhale
With strong core, slowly return your spine to vertical from bottom to top.

❯ Listen to your body, only performing movement that feels comfortable.

❯ Maintain abdominal connection, supporting spine during extension.

❯ Keep shoulder blades sliding back and down.

❯ Extend evenly through spine, as far as feels comfortable.

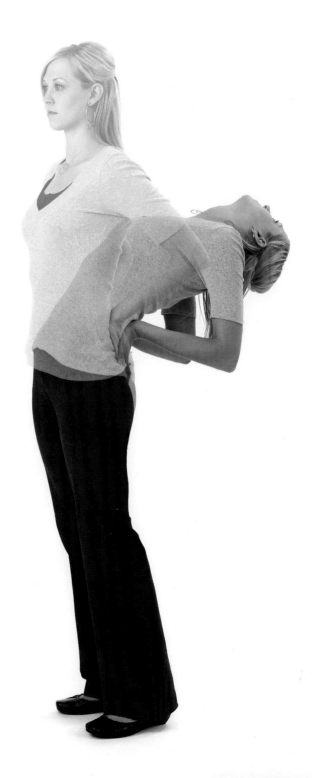

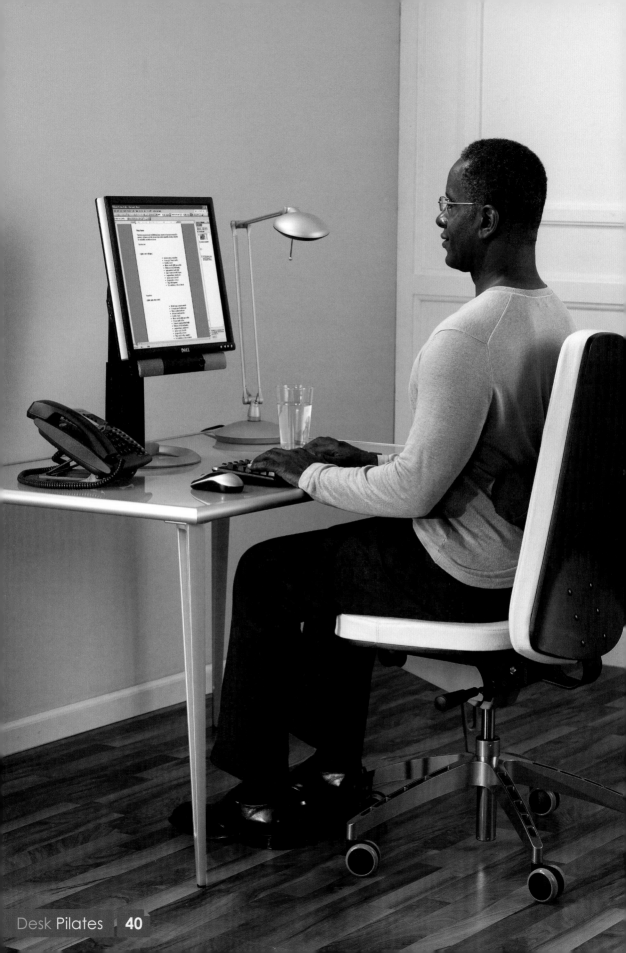

Living Pilates
at Your Desk

Integrate the essentials of Pilates to focus on the quality of each moment throughout your day—breathe fully, keep your center strong, and reconnect your body and your brain.

Be mindful to —
> Align your spine in neutral
> Breathe deeply, exhaling fully
> Engage abdominals
> Lengthen through your spine
> Widen across your chest
> Relax neck and shoulders

Remember that your own body awareness is the most important factor for your comfort and alignment. While looking at your desk space and your chair, think about how you can best apply Pilates principles and maintain your optimal healthy posture throughout your day. Intermittently perform self-checks by asking yourself the following questions.

Are you breathing deeply to reduce muscle tension and improve your mental focus?
Do you vary activities and plan movement breaks at least hourly during your day?
Are you walking often, at least a few steps to your water cooler, printer, copier, or fax?
When at your desk, are your tasks positioned directly in front of you?

Is your chair the right height and size for you?
Do you sit with your bottom all the way to the back of the chair seat, with your thighs fully supported, and comfortable space for the backs of your knees?
Are your hips level with or slightly higher than your knees?
Do your feet rest comfortably on the floor or on a footrest?

Is your weight evenly distributed on both sit bones?
Are you sitting with your pelvis and spine in neutral alignment?
Would lumbar support help to maintain the curve in your low back?
When leaning forward, do you hinge from your hips, keeping your spine lengthened?

Are your neck and shoulders free from tension?
When talking on the phone, are your head and neck neutral?
If using armrests, are your forearms supported at elbow height and comfortably close to your body?

When using a computer, is it positioned right in front of you?
Is the mouse and keyboard positioned to keep your shoulders relaxed, your elbows relaxed and open at your sides, your forearms parallel to the floor, and your wrists neutral?
Do you sometimes try challenging your body and brain with non-dominant hand mouse use?

Does the height of your computer screen allow a comfortable, relaxed gaze?
Do you blink your eyes frequently, and every 20 minutes look away from the screen out a window or at an object 20 feet away, for at least 20 seconds?

Using a Laptop

Your body awareness remains crucial during laptop computer use. Laptops are wonderfully convenient, efficient, and portable, however they are not as adjustable as desktop computers for comfortable, consistent, everyday use.

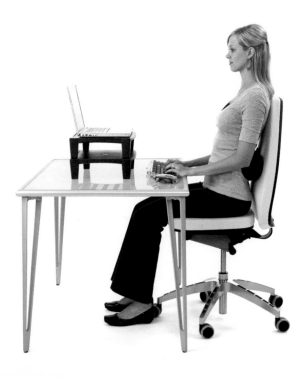

Occasional use —

> Neck near neutral, tension free
> Screen angled for neck comfort
> Shoulders relaxed
> Elbows relaxed, slightly open at sides
> Wrists neutral while keyboarding
> Laptop positioned comfortably
> Chair reclined back to 110 degrees
> Lengthened spine, natural curves
> Lumbar support, if needed
> Sitting evenly on sit bones
> Thighs fully supported
> Feet comfortably on floor or footrest

Frequent use —

> Elevate laptop on monitor pedestal
> Screen positioned for relaxed gaze
> External keyboard and mouse
> Neck neutral and tension free
> Shoulders relaxed
> Elbows relaxed, slightly open at sides
> Forearms near parallel to floor
> If armrests, supporting at desk height
> Wrists neutral while keyboarding
> Lengthened spine, natural curves
> Lumbar support, if needed
> Sitting evenly on sit bones
> Thighs parallel to floor, supported
> Feet comfortably on floor or footrest

Sitting Actively

Replacing your chair with an exercise ball for part of the day promotes dynamic sitting that actively engages your body's core muscles, as well as your hips, legs, knees, ankles, and feet. The unstable surface gently challenges your balance and inherently requires your body and mind to work together while sitting. The seated *Desk Pilates* exercises can be effectively performed while sitting on an exercise ball.

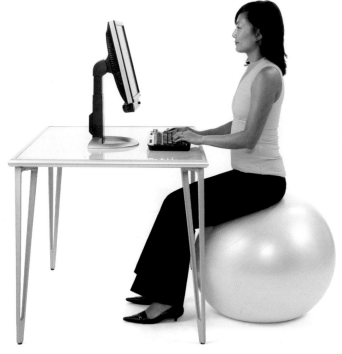

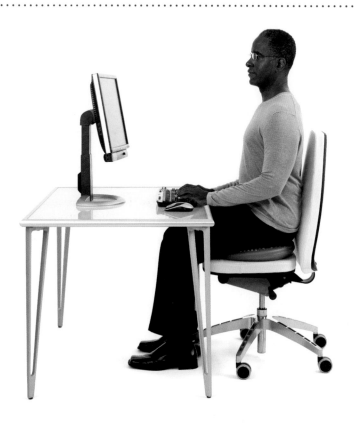

Sitting on an inflatable disc also activates your core muscles for optimal postural alignment and provides an additional core challenge during *Desk Pilates* exercises. The disc easily moves from one chair to another, or can also be used as a footrest to encourage healthy foot, ankle, and leg movements during sitting.

Applying
Desk Pilates

At a glance, these small photos reference each *Desk Pilates* exercise. By design, your body requires a variety of movements throughout each day. Remember to shift your positions and change your activities frequently, incorporating a few moments of walking and Pilates exercise breaks.

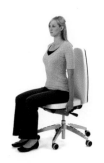

Spine Lengthening
page 18

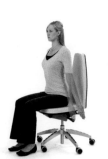

Hundred
page 19

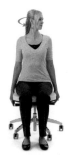

Neck Turn
page 20

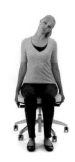

Neck Side Bend
page 21

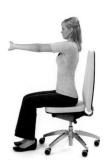

Shoulder Reach
page 22

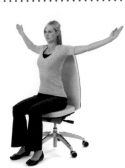

Arm Circles
page 23

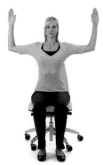

Open Elbows
page 24

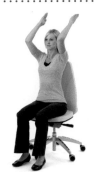

Elbow Reach
page 25

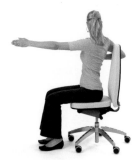

Spine Twist
page 26

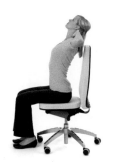

Sternum Lift
page 27

Be mindful to —
❯ Align spine in neutral
❯ Breathe deeply, exhaling fully
❯ Engage abdominals
❯ Lengthen through your spine
❯ Widen across your chest
❯ Relax your neck and shoulders

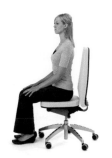

Gluteal Squeeze
page 28

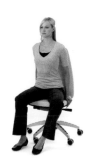

Knee Drop
page 29

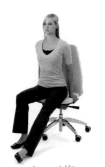

Leg Lift
page 30

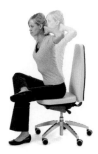

Hip Hinge
page 31

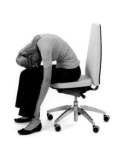

Spine Stretch Forward
page 32

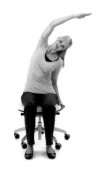

Mermaid
page 33

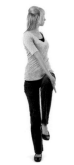

Standing Criss-Cross
page 34

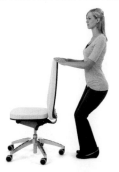

Bend and Stretch
page 35

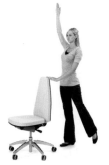

Swimming
page 36

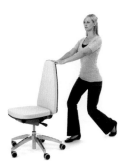

Heel Lift & Lower
page 37

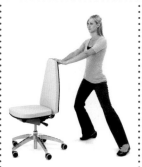

Skating
page 38

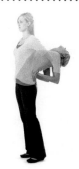

Swan Dive
page 39

Pilates Resources

OPTP
3800 Annapolis Lane, Suite 165
Minneapolis, MN 55447
800.367.7393
www.optp.com

Stott Pilates
2200 Younge Street, #1402
Toronto, Ontario M4S 2C6
Canada
800.910.0001
www.stottpilates.com

Pilates Method Alliance
2631 Lincoln Avenue
Miami, FL 33133
305.573.4946
866.573.4945
www.pilatesmethodalliance.org

About the author

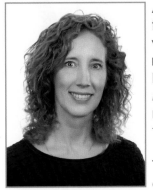

Angela Kneale, OTR, is a 1994 summa cum laude graduate from the College of St. Catherine in St. Paul, Minnesota, who has achieved full certification from internationally recognized Stott Pilates. She is the author of Stretch Out Strap Pilates Essentials, Pro-Roller Pilates Essentials and Pro-Roller Massage Essentials, and she specializes in the integration of movement, breathing, postural alignment, and relaxation techniques for optimal health and wellness.

Tremendous gratitude is extended to her family and friends, especially sons Quinn and Zane Sullivan, who continually inspire learning, love, and laughter; James E. Mullen, M.D., and many professional colleagues and clients whose experiences and wisdom nurture additional learning, growth, and sharing.

Special thanks to her parents, Collan Kneale and Janet Kneale Toigo.